Felipe Reyes

COMMUNITY NURSING ELEMENTS

Felipe Reyes

COMMUNITY NURSING ELEMENTS

Quality community nursing care

ScienciaScripts

Imprint

Any brand names and product names mentioned in this book are subject to trademark, brand or patent protection and are trademarks or registered trademarks of their respective holders. The use of brand names, product names, common names, trade names, product descriptions etc. even without a particular marking in this work is in no way to be construed to mean that such names may be regarded as unrestricted in respect of trademark and brand protection legislation and could thus be used by anyone.

Cover image: www.ingimage.com

This book is a translation from the original published under ISBN 978-620-3-03277-2.

Publisher:
Sciencia Scripts
is a trademark of
Dodo Books Indian Ocean Ltd. and OmniScriptum S.R.L publishing group

120 High Road, East Finchley, London, N2 9ED, United Kingdom
Str. Armeneasca 28/1, office 1, Chisinau MD-2012, Republic of Moldova, Europe
Managing Directors: Ieva Konstantinova, Victoria Ursu
info@omniscriptum.com

Printed at: see last page
ISBN: 978-620-3-12055-4

ELEMENTS OF COMMUNITY NURSING

Author: Tania Felipe

Reyes Graduate in

Nursing

1st Grade Community Nurse Specialist

Assistant Professor at the Faculty of Medical Sciences of Sancti Spiritus Cuba.

Collaborators

Msc Maria Elena Pacheco Sosa Ing.

Ms.C Benigno Leyva de la Cruz Esp.

DEDICATORY

This book is dedicated to nursing professionals working in primary health care, nursing students and teachers.

PREFACE

The diversity of community health issues was the reason for the elaboration of this text whose purpose is to unify contents of importance for the community professional as a guide for his or her daily work. The book is intended for all nursing students, teachers and professionals who work in primary health care. It describes in a dynamic and entertaining way the different work algorithms in community work.

For its preparation, national and international bibliographical reviews have been carried out, extracting the useful aspects for the community work. Taking into account methodological aspects of the contents for the affordable assimilation of these contents.

The use of this text favors the organized work of the nurse with community assignment and the preparation of a competent professional for the performance of community work.

INDEX

CHAPTER 1: EMERGENCE OF COMMUNITY NURSING

The Community Nursing was born with the creation of the Ministry of Health and Social Assistance and valuing the family as a work unit, this situation determined that each nurse was assigned a certain number of families and communities in her charge. The community infirmary is the part of the infirmary that develops and applies in an integral way, within the framework of public health, the care of the individual, the family and the community in health and illness. Community nursing is a synthesis of nursing practice and public health applied to promote and preserve the health of the population. The nature of this practice is general and covers many aspects. It is continuous and contributes to improving the health of the population as a whole. Nursing care in the community goes back to the knowledge of life itself and the notion of human survival, focusing on the health needs of the population, throughout the life of the individual. Community Nursing is the part of nursing that develops and applies in an integral manner the care of families and communities in the unstable balance of health illness. It specifically contributes to individuals, families and communities acquiring skills, habits and behaviors that promote self-care within the framework of primary health care, which includes promotion, protection, recovery, prevention and rehabilitation of health.

Health problems and needs must be addressed from a quality and interdisciplinary perspective. Community nursing must be an advocate for values that contribute to maintaining greater solidarity and social justice, and equal opportunities. The community nurse should monitor health in the community as a whole and determine the impact of their actions on groups or sets of groups served in relation to the total community and its level of health. The community nurse redirects and trains individuals, families and communities to care for themselves and is able to transform dependency into self-care.

It has its antecedents in the English Health Movement of the 19th century, after the Chadwick report (1837)

-William Rathbone and Florence Nightingale

-The health visitor system was developed in the 20th century.

-It also extended to other countries from Europe to the United States leading to the creation of schools.

1.1 Mission and vision

The vision of the community nurse before society is expressed as an integral service in all the assistance processes with the vision of the nursing process as a work tool and with assistance practice based on scientific evidence.

The mission is to help individuals, families and communities determine and achieve their physical, mental and social potential and realize it within the environment in which they live and work.

1.2 Community Nurse Roles

The personnel who assist the community environment and who are endowed with all the ethical and moral principles that the profession requires, develop professional skills that facilitate the best development of the assigned task and have the responsibility to go through all the activities entrusted to the nursing professional.

- Assistance: This refers to the work that is done in the health institution and the work that is done in the community, pursuing the preventive, curative and rehabilitation of individuals, families and the community.

- Teacher: The health professional carries out health promotion activities using methodological aspects that make the understanding of the different topics possible, as well as collaborating in the training of the new generation.

- Administration: The nursing professional performs administrative control of equipment, accessories and medications that are under his custody for patient care, as well as coordinates activities of the health team.

- Researcher: In order to raise the quality of patient care, the nursing professional must be updated on health and care issues and therefore it is necessary that they are incorporated into the conduct of research.

the annual health situation analysis is one of the most important tools for the main epidemiological investigations carried out by community care personnel and which constitute an indissoluble tool for community work.

1.3 Characteristics of community care

The community attention to achieve the proposed purpose or objective must bring together a number of qualities that make the work is done optimally, involving different sectors that from their radius of action provide benefits for the implementation of actions aimed at the same end as they are:

- Integral
- Integrator
- Continuous and permanent
- Activate
- Accessible
- Multidisciplinary
- Participative
- Programmed
- Evaluable
- Teacher
- Researcher

CHAPTER 2: CROSS-CULTURAL NURSING

The relationship of culture with nursing and with anthropology is long and extensive. Each individual internalizes and applies the care according to his/her culture, that is to say, according to his/her customs, values, beliefs, and since the beginning of the world, these techniques have somehow served as a means of survival. This situation is confirmed with the development of cross-cultural nursing where cultural competence is considered a necessary condition for nursing care in all patients.

Nurses must be careful to discern with respect to personal cultural values and beliefs and separate them from the values and beliefs of the patients they are dealing with. In order to provide culturally sensitive care, nurses must remember that each individual is unique and is the product of customary beliefs, values passed on from one generation to the next. Becoming aware and accepting cultural differences is an exercise that compromises the actions of the nurse. We should not fall into paternalistic behavior, nor, on the contrary, should we treat the person from another culture as we would any other person, respecting individual differences and focusing on the quality of the humanized service we are providing. The area of cross-cultural nursing means fleeing from stereotypes and overcoming prejudices in order to establish an effective relationship with the user, accepting cultural differences.

2.1 Concept of cross-cultural nursing

It is based on an ideology as a way of focusing care towards cultural consideration in its practice, as Lenninger stated it is no more than providing care that is coherent with the culture in order to give quality to it, and for this, the individual culture must be known in order to be applied. Nursing personnel with cross-cultural training must take into account cultural beliefs, care behaviors and values of individuals in an individualized way, as well as families and different social groups in their charge to provide effective, satisfactory and coherent care with the objective of developing a body of humanized and scientific knowledge to provide a culturally specific and universal nursing practice.

Cross-Cultural Nursing: Nurses who are trained in cross-cultural nursing and whose job it is to develop the knowledge and practice of cross-cultural nursing are refiere

Cross-cultural nursing : Nurses using medical or applied anthropological concepts are refiere authorized to develop cross-cultural nursing theory and research-based practice.

2.2 Ethical principles of the nursing professional in transculturation

Compliance with ethical nursing principles is of vital importance to achieve the objectives proposed by the community nurse.

1. Beneficence: benevolence or non-maleficence, the ethical principle of doing good and avoiding harm or evil to your self or to society. Acting benevolently means helping others to obtain what is beneficial to them, or which promotes their well-being, by reducing the evil risks, which may cause them physical or psychological harm.

2. Autonomy: ethical principle that advocates the individual freedom that each person has to determine their own actions, according to their choice. Respecting people as autonomous individuals means recognizing their decisions, made in accordance with their personal values and convictions. One of the problems in the application of the principle of autonomy in nursing care is that the patient may present different levels of capacity to make an autonomous decision, depending on his/her internal limitations (mental aptitude, level of consciousness, age or health condition) or external ones (hospital environment, availability of existing resources, amount of information provided for making an informed decision, among others).

3. Justice: Once the ways of practicing charity have been determined, the nurse needs to be concerned with how to distribute these benefits or resources among his or her patients as the disposition of his or her t i e m p o and care among the various patients according to the needs that arise. Justice is the principle of being equitable or fair, that is, equal treatment among equals and differential treatment among unequals, according to individual need. This ignores the fact that people with the same health needs should receive the same quantity and quality of services and resources. The principle of justice is closely related to the principles of fidelity and truthfulness.

4. Loyalty: principle of creating trust between the professional and the patient. It is, in fact, an obligation or commitment to be faithful in the relationship with the patient, in which the nurse must make promises and maintain reliability. The patient's expectation is that the professionals will follow through on the words given. Only in exceptional circumstances, when the benefits of breaking the promise are greater than its maintenance, can the promise be broken. Trust is the basis for spontaneous confidence, and facts revealed in confidence are part of the professional secret of the nurse.

5. Truthfulness: ethical principle of always telling the truth, not lying and not deceiving patients. In many cultures, truthfulness has been considered the basis for establishing and maintaining trust between individuals. An example of such a variation woul d be on the amount of information to be provided in relation to diagnosis and treatment. Thus, it may be difficult to develop a form to obtain the consent of the patient, who has not been informed of his or her diagnosis.

The professional must assess the importance to the participant of knowing his or her diagnosis in relation to the intended treatment or care.

6. Confidentiality: ethical principle to safeguard the personal information obtained during the exercise of their function as a nurse and to maintain the character of professional secrecy of this information, not communicating to anyone the personal confidences made by the patients

Ethics and values are unavoidable principles that must characterize the professionals of the Nursing, which demands respect, dignity to the life, quality efficiency, beneficence, veracity, justice towards the patient to whom the care is granted.

2.3 Nursing Theory that supports the transculturation of community care nurses

Madeleine Leininger

"Cultural care: theory of diversity and universality"

Leininger, the founder of cross-cultural nursing and a leader in the theory of care for people, was the first college-educated professional nurse to earn an award in cultural and social anthropology. She was born in Sutton, Nebraska and began her career as a nurse after graduating from St. Anthony's Denver School o f Nursing.

Theoretical sources

Leininger drew on the discipline of anthropology and nursing definió cross-cultural nursing as a major area of nursing that focuses on the comparative study and analysis of different cultures and subcultures of the world with respect to values about care, expression and beliefs about health and illness, and modeling of behavior, whose purpose is to conceive of a científico and humanistic knowledge to provide a nursing practice específicos for culture and a universal nursing care practice of culture.

Cross-Cultural Nursing goes beyond knowledge and uses the knowledge of cultural nursing to practice culturally congruent and responsible care

Leininger states that over time there will be a new type of nursing practice that will reflejará different types of nursing, which will be definirán and culture-based and will be específicos to guide nursing care for individuals, families, groups and institutions. Afirma that culture and care are the broadest means of conceptualizing and understanding people this knowledge is essential to nursing education and practice

Leininger defiende which, just like nursing is significativa for patients and nurses all over the world the knowledge of cross-cultural nursing and its competencies will be indispensable to guide the decisions and actions of nurses and thus obtain good results and eficaces able to apply general concepts principles and practices of cross-cultural nursing created by the cross-cultural nursing specialists on the other hand Leinninger defiende and promotes a new and different theory, and not the traditional theory of nursing, which is normally define as a set of concepts related to each other in a logical way and hypothetical propositions that can be proved to fin to explain or predict a fact, phenomenon or situation. Instead, Leininger defiende theory as the systematic and creative discovery of knowledge of a field of interest or a phenomenon that seems relevant to understand or explain unknown phenomena.

Leininger, created the theory of diversity and universality of cultural nursing care, which is based on the belief that people from different cultures can inform and guide professionals and thus be able to receive the type of health care they want and need from these professionals. Cultures represent the systematized models of their lives and the values of the people who influyen in their decisions and actions. Therefore, the theory is focused for nurses to discover and acquire the knowledge about the world of the patient and for them to make use of their internal points of view, their knowledge.

CHAPTER 3: THE HOME VISIT

The home visit is the set of social and health activities provided at home to people. This attention allows to detect, to value, to support and to control the problems of health of the individual and the family, harnessing the autonomy and improving the quality of life of the people, is considered the basic activity of the nurse in the sense of solving the problems of health and crisis of the individual, the family and the community, allowing to make actions of promotion and prevention of health to obtain styles of healthy lives, allows the healing, rehabilitation and incorporation to the society. The home visit is a strategy of delivery of health services at home for families within the framework of a plan of action defined by the health team, allowing health interventions in the context of people's lives.

3.1 Objectives

1- The objective of the home visit is to verify the composition of the family nucleus, the socio-economic level of the individual, the distribution of social spaces, personal and family behavior, family health and relevant aspects to be evaluated since they directly impact the population in their care, and to contribute to raising the quality of life through integrated and coordinated actions of health promotion, prevention and rehabilitation.

2- To promote the actions of the environment and family ties that favor the biopsychosocial development of the population.

3- Extend care coverage to all members of the family group.

4- Improve the use of available resources through the application of protocols according to age groups, pathologies and needs.

3.2 Structure or stages

Planning: This is done by the health team, coordinating date, time and objective.

Introduction: Explain to the family the objective of the visit, being important the rapor that should be created by the nurse in order to achieve a climate of trust and security between nurse, family, patient.

Development: It is divided for its better development in 3 stages. We work on the aspects that motivated the visit.

1- Walk through the home: Risk factors are identified, family functioning test (FF-SIL test) is performed

2- General physical examination of the individual

3- Observation of environmental hygiene risks in the community.

Conclusions: It is the summary of the most important aspects, elaborating a plan of action that the family must follow in the absence of the nurse, leaving recommendations and coordinating the next visit.

The estimated time of the home visit will depend on the family situation and the objectives set. It should take approximately 20 or 30 minutes.

Evaluation of the home visit: An analysis is made by the members of the team and health to evaluate the fulfillment of the proposed objectives.

Types of home visits

- First contact: it is done for the first time in the house, it arises from an initial intervention plan and is done to establish the first contact.

- Follow-up visit: They are part of an intervention plan and evaluation of the objectives set.

- Epidemiological visit: Destined to make an epidemiological investigation of a pathology that is under surveillance.

- Rescue or summoning of patients: You go home to make an appointment for a specific health task or to find out about the absence of an appointment.

- Unsuccessful visit: When you go home and can't get in touch with the family

Advantages of the home visit

✓ Allows the family to be observed in its environmental and social environment

✓ The family actively participates

✓ It allows the nurse to be aware of the social environmental characteristics of the families in her care

Qualities of the human resource

✓ Training and education

✓ Professional experience

✓ Ability to relate

✓ Providing relevant information at the right time

✓ Ability to develop trusting relationships with family members, interest and commitment to the task

3.3 Requirements for an effective visit

The family environment requires privacy on the part of its members so the nursing professional has the obligation to establish guidelines of behavior, ethical elements and professional development that allow him/her to efficiently carry out this community practice.

- Family or individual needs: Working with the felt needs of the population allows the professional to have accessibility to the family and the achievement of the objectives.

- Pathological history: The nursing staff, if they visit for the first time, should make an extensive anamnesis, emphasizing family and personal pathological history that will allow them to work with the risk factors and thus avoid triggering the disease.

- Accommodation conditions: The conditions for the effective visit must be created in advance e.g. domestic animals must be protected to avoid injury to health personnel, rooms must be lit and ventilated, and a room must be available for the physical examination and the conclusions of the visit.

- Health facilities and cultural environment. The health staff will create a favorable rapport environment to facilitate family exchange and to ensure that the interview and other community procedures are conducted in a fruitful manner.

3.4 Case technique

Through the use of the briefcase the nurse provides indirect teaching, the family observes carefully the information provided, specific equipment and materials are used, serving as motivation at the same time.

Case technique

Objectives: To bring basic equipment to provide nursing care at home or elsewhere, according to need.

Provide nursing care, including techniques and demonstrations. Procedure:

Before leaving for the field, prepare the briefcase according to the planificación of your home visit and probable situations that could arise, according to the family, school, kindergarten, company, etc. to visit. In order to carry out a home visit eficaz you must take into account that you will be given a suitable briefcase with the necessary items for the visit.

Through the use of the briefcase, the nurse provides indirect instruction; the family carefully observes the information provided, and equipment and materials are used específicos.

Contents of the case:

Its content is valid, except for the transfer of biological products, which must be placed in the areas recommended in the universal vaccination program.

Instrumental

- Heavy duty clamp (Rochester)

Team

- Sterile and non-sterile test tube in quantity suficiente

- Clinical rectal or axillary thermometer

- Baumanometer

- Pinard Stethoscope

- Portfolio with home visit request forms and educational material.

Consumption material

Basic Equipment:1 case

1 bottle with alcohol (60 to 100cc)

1 bottle with alcohol dry hand washing gel if necessary 3 ampoules

of serum fisiológico of 20cc

1 bottle with liquid soap

1 scissors

3 disposable tongue depressors

1 bottle with dry cotton swabs (large and small) Nova towel 1 plastic bib 1 nylon 0.50 cm x 0.50 cm

1 paper of 0.50 cm x 0.50 cm (type kraft or white paper, not printed) Paper or plastic waste bags.

1 measuring cup

Non-sterile disposable gloves

1 esfigmomanómetro with

stethoscope 1 flashlight

1 thermometer

1 small clean kidney (to place the thermometer)

1 monofilamento (piece of fishing line)

1 small file cabinet with set of educational materials

According to the need, material will be added to the basic equipment to perform techniques específicas, such as cures, taking urine and blood tests at home, material for DSM stimulation, weight, etc.

Basic technique for the use of the

case Steps:

1. Choose a flat, resistant, safe and comfortable place; hold the wallet and the case with one hand: take out the plastic frame from between the fins and the cover and spread it over the chosen place

2. Place the case on a paper field on the left side.

3. Wash your hands with water or ask the family for a container of clean water.

4. Dry your m a n s with the p ap e ly towel and   throw it away in the waste bag.

5. Open the case.

6. Remove the material and equipment that you need from the case and   place it in a clean field.

7. It performs the necessary activities and procedures by carrying them out in an orderly manner.

8. Make the necessary notes.

9. Store material and equipment in the case in an orderly manner.

10. Disposal   the bag   de d es ec h o sel material used during procedures as well as the paper field.

11. It closes the case perfectly.

Case for home visit of infirmary, specially destined to transport medical material, being of the type constituted by a prismatic body (2), equipped with blocks of support (3) in its inferior base (4), as well as of a handle (5), characterized by the fact that the mentioned one.

CHAPTER 4: PALLIATIVE CARE FOR PATIENTS IN THE COMMUNITY

Palliative care in the home allows people to remain in their own homes for care at the end of their lives. At these times, families require outside help. Therefore, many families choose caregivers with experience in palliative nursing and care. Nursing staff from hospice care assume roles ranging from pain management and symptom control to assessing coping mechanisms for both the patient and the family and providing them with the resources available for their care.

According to the WHO palliative care is appropriate for the patient with advanced and progressive disease where the control of pain and other symptoms, as well as psychosocial and spiritual aspects become more important.

In the integral attention to the patient in advanced phase of the disease in his residence. It has great advantages and some disadvantages for the patient and for the family. It is the essence of palliative care and with well-configured equipment it is possible to give good quality of life and dignified death to patients with advanced terminal illness.

Advantages for the patient

He maintains his social and family role, disposes of his time and distributes it, maintains his intimacy and his occupational activities for the patient and the family, is in a familiar environment, has the affection of his family and it has been proven that there is an increase in the quality of life with respect to hospitalized patients.

Benefits for the family

Familiar environment, ease of movement, time, satisfaction with active participation in care, facilitation of the grieving process, respect for the patient's will.

4.1 Nursing theory that supports the palliative work of the nursing professional in the community

Dorothea Orem's general theory is composed of 3 related theories: Theory of self-care

Theory of self-care deficit Theory

of nursing systems Other theories

such as:

Jean Watson's theory

Florence Nightingale's

Theory Calista Roy's Theory

4.2 Palliative Care Objectives

The goal of palliative care is to achieve the best quality of life for the patient and his or her family, to obtain a dignified death. Palliative care treatments are not mutually exclusive, but rather a matter of emphasis.

4.3 Hospice patient's needs for palliative care

Taking into account the basic needs for the conservation of life and the hierarchical elements of the Kalish pyramid, the community nurse will identify in each patient which are the needs that are appearing in each stage of the palliative care, as well as the technical elements that each need must fulfill in order to achieve the goals set, we refer to the following needs:

❖ Hygiene, rest and sleep needs

❖ Nutritional needs

❖ Urinary elimination needs

❖ Intestinal elimination needs.

❖ Oxygen needs

❖ Need for security and self-esteem.

4.4 Bed Bath Procedure

Bath in shower). This is the bath that is done under running water, with the help of the nursing staff, unless contraindicated by the doctor.

Objectives:

- Maintain personal hygiene.
- facilitate the transfer.
- Activate peripheral circulation and exercise the patient's muscles and limbs.

-      Establish a good relationship with the patient.

- Observe the patient's general condition or pathological signs of skin.
- To provide well-being and

comfort. Precautions:

- Measuring vital signs before bathing

- Protect the patient from accidents and colds.

- Make sure the water temperature is adequate.

- Avoid prolonged bathing

- Supplying all the necessary material

- Helps the patient return to his unit

Material

- Bench or chair.

- Patient's wardrobe.

- Large and small towel.

- Personal hygiene items, lotion, deodorant, shampoo.

Procedure:

- Evaluate vital signs.

- To arrange the conditions to carry out the bath.

- Orient the patient to urinate.

- Take the patient to the bathroom and adjust the ventilation.

- Help the patient get undressed and maintain their privacy.

- Make everything easy for the patient to bathe by himself, if he is in condition to do so, otherwise, it must be done by the nurse in a quick way to avoid body cooling.

- Start the bath on the face then the head, chest, upper extremities, back, abdomen, lower extremities, genitals and buttocks.

- provide the towel to dry or help you, if necessary.

- It helps the patient to get dressed and go back to the unit.

Bathing in the riverbed. It consists of cleaning the skin with soap and water, in the patient who is partially or totally dependent.

Procedure. Place

the paraban.

Offer wedge or potty, if the patient desires it.

- Wash your hands and lower the Fowler (if not contraindicated).

- Remove the patient's clothing while maintaining their privacy.

- Keep the patient covered with the sheet up to the shoulders.

- Place the clothes on the premises in the unwashed clothes cart that should be at the foot of the bed

- Arrange and check the water temperature.

-Place a cloth in the container to be used for washing the patient and another cloth in the container to be used for rinsing.

- Place the rinsing cloth in the shape of a glove so that the extremities of the fingers are protected, in order to avoid hurting the skin with the nails.

- Soap the face, ears and neck, avoid soap entering the eye if there is an eye condition, should be done before the eye wash

- Rinse and dry in the same way as soap.

- Lower the sheet to the pubic region.

- Rinse the thorax insisting on infra-mammary folds, the abdomen and both the upper limbs (emphasizing the armpits, elbow folds and interdigital spaces), rinse and dry in the same order.

- Cover the patient's chest.

- Place the patient in a lateral position to soap, rinse and dry the cervical region up to the buttocks.

- Turn the patient (dorsal decubitus) and keep the chest covered.

- Uncover the lower limbs and rinse both thighs and legs down to the ankles. Wash and dry.

- Soap both feet, insist on interdigital spaces, rinse and dry.

Technique for dressing and undressing

Sick

Dressing - Covering the body with

clothing.

Wardrobe. Define the hors d'oeuvres that serve to cover the body from the hygienic point of view.

Clothing should be a poor heat conductor so that thermal changes with the outside environment are gradual to conserve and maintain body heat in winter and the warmer season to avoid outside temperature.

Objective:

- Maintain personal hygiene, cover the body and promote patient comfort.

Precautions:

-Avoid drafts Cautions

Have all the necessary material ready.

Keep in mind the patient's state of consciousness. -Use the size that best matches the patient's physical constitution.

- When it comes to dressing the patient, do it first because of the wound or limited area.

-The clothes must be without wrinkles.

-Applying body mechanics.

Material

-Pyjamas or evening shirt.

-Disordered laundry basket or cart.

-Biombo (if

necessary).

Procedure:

- Place the paraban (if necessary).

- Place the patient in a seated or semi-seated position, if his condition allows it.

- Discover the sleeve of the pajamas or shirt, first removing one arm at a time.

-I wear the same arm with pajamas or shirt.

- Proceed in the same manner for the other senior member.

-Button the shirt.

-Remove the top sheet and open it to fit into your pajamas.

-Orient the patient to bend the legs and lift the buttocks, if their situation allows it.

-Drop your pants and remove them.

-Place the pants neatly in the same way (first lower limb, then the other.

4.5 Morning and afternoon care procedure

Morning care: this is the care given to disabled patients, partially or totally in the early morning hours.

Objectives:
-Clean, refresh and relax the patient.

-Arrange the patient for the little lunch.

-Provide aesthetics.

-Educate the patient on hygienic aspects,
-Eliminate the accumulation of fat on the skin of the face, eye and nasal secretions.

Precautions:

-Maintain patient privacy.

-Use water at an appropriate temperature, according to the patient's habits.

Afternoon care: This is the care given to the partially or totally disabled patient at the end of the afternoon.

Objective:

-To satisfy the physical and psychological needs of the patient to promote a restful sleep.

Precautions:

-Maintain patient privacy.

-Do not massage the legs to avoid embolism.

-To observe the state of the skin and the sacral region, before giving the massage (strengthening, cracks, other signs or damage).

-Check dressings, ligatures and anti-embolism stockings, alter or adjust.

4.6 Procedure for feeding a patient with palliative care

Nasogastric Intubation: is the introduction of a tube through the nostrils or from the mouth to the stomach.

Objectives:

1. Establish the medical diagnosis.

2. Apply therapeutic measures.

3. Feed the patient who cannot do it spontaneously.

4. Establish a means of draining the gastric content and extracting gases.

5. Preventing vomiting and abdominal distension

Precautions:

1) Have all the necessary material ready.

2) Keep in mind the patient's state of consciousness.

3) Use the size that best matches the patient's physical constitution.

Place the patient in a semi-seated position if possible; the patient is unconscious in the Trendelenburg position, leaning on the left side in a ventral position. This position prevents unpleasant aspiration.

4) Moisten the probe with distilled water or saline solution, avoiding dripping, never with fatty substances, to avoid irritating the mucous membranes and rough aspiration.

5) Ask the patient why the nostril is breathing better, and pass the probe through the one that has the most difficulty.

6) If the individual presents any nasal alteration, such as a deviated septum, that prevents the probe from passing through the mouth, introduce it through the mouth after having removed the dental prosthesis.

7) If the person is unconscious, tilt the chin to the chest to close the trachea and push the tube between breaths to make sure it did not stop the trachea

8) Watch for signs of entry into the windpipe, drowning or difficult breathing in a conscious person and cyanosis in an unconscious or non-reflexed cough. If these signs are present, immediately remove the tube, allow the patient to rest and try again.

9) To check the correct positioning of the probe, never insert the end of the probe in the water. If the probe is in the trachea, the patient may inhale water; and in any case, the absence of bubbles does not confirm correct placement, because the probe may be swollen in the trachea or in the esophagus.

10) Check that the tube is in the stomach.

11) Measuring gastric content

Material:

1) Tray or side table.

2) Gastric probe (Latex, silicone, with balloon

3) Towel, cloth, or

receipt. Feeding probe

Feeding probe: It is the introduction of liquid or melted food through a tube that passes through the nose or mouth to the stomach.

Objective:

Maintain proper patient nutritional status

Precautions:

Ensure the hygienic condition of the oral and nasal cavities.

Aspirate before administering food and observe the characteristics of the substances extracted.

If the aspirated content is greater than 100 ml, do not feed the patient and inform the doctor.

Measure the amount of food and water administered, supplying them at an adequate temperature.

Gravity food management

Alter the tube with the current norms of hygiene and epidemiology, to avoid damage to the hydrochloric acid in the stomach and cause an unnecessary response.

Avoid sudden movements that may cause the patient to vomit, once the food has been given

Material

Gastric probe (Levine, among

others). Towel, washcloth, or

receipt.

Garbage cans. Glass

with water.

Adhesive, edge to fix the

probe. Scissors.

Spatulas.

Compres

ses.

Paper towels or napkin.

Stethoscope.

20 ml syringe, feeding syringe, funnel or disposable feeding bag

Clamp mounted.

Container with food

Container with water

Bladder catheterization procedure for patients with difficulty in urination
Elimination would pay for palliative care

Bladder catheterization is the introduction of a tube or catheter through the meatus
and urethral canal into the bladder.

Objectives:

Bladder emptying.

To determine if urine deficit is caused by urinary retention obstruction, or anuria.

Obtain urine samples for the study.

Emptying the bladder before major surgery to avoid surgical trauma at the organ level and the patient urinating in the operating room to cause sphincter relaxation

Precautions:

Cleanse the genitals to reduce bacteria to that level and avoid being dragged into the bladder.

Do not force the catheter through, to avoid trauma to the urethra, keep in mind the caliber of the catheters for the type of urethra;

Ask the patient to cough during insertion, as this will make it easier to insert the tube.

After completing the procedure, the uncircumcised man should be careful to push the foreskin over the glans.

In the case of the Foley probe, fix it with saline solution (no air, no glucose solutions).

If the catheter remains stationary, periodically clamp it to regain bladder tone.

If the urine is retained, allow up to 400 ml every 30 minutes, allow 200 ml to escape to avoid rapid urine stagnation.

Change of probes according to service

standards. Team

Compresses.

Waste container.

Sterile syringe with physiological

serum Tape (remains permanent).

Scissors (remains permanent).

Collector bag (remains

permanent). Stop (if necessary).

Intestinal elimination procedure in a patient with palliative care

Emollient Enemas. When there is severe constipation, painful anal disorder or irritation of the intestinal mucosa a fatty enema can be dated. The oil acts mainly as a lubricant to facilitate evacuation. Various oils can be used, such as mineral, oil, cotton seed and others. The amount used is small, generally 150 to 200 ml and usually the patient is asked to retain the enema for about 1 H. Many times, after a retention enema, a cleansing enema is indicated.

Precautions:

o Administer cleansing enema beforehand, to keep the colon free of feces.
o Hold it 10-20 M.
o Apply lubricant in the anal and perianal region and in the internal part of the thighs will be performed anthelmintic enema.
o Retention Enemas should be scheduled before meals, because a full stomach can stimulate peristalsis.
o Oil retention enema should not be administered before cleansing enema, but to do it 1 hour after the fatty enema, recommends that it be of soap and water to help expel the stool completely softened.
o In anti-parasitic enemas, once administered, you must then proceed with a cleansing enema.
o If the sphincter is not functional, place a rectal probe with a balloon.
o Complications can occur from the enema that is retained.

Material:

o General enema equipment.
o He added the indicated medication, gloves and a syringe to measure the medication, if necessary.

Procedure for administering oxygen in a patient who is undergoing palliative care.

Oxygen by nasal moustache

Metal support. Metal fixation with a fork with two recessed hooks (which allow the oxygen bill), slightly concave to be placed in the nostrils.

Plastic fork. Hollow plastic attachment with two short, straight extensions that can be perfectly attached to the nose.

Objective: To apply oxygen therapy with a mustache when the patient has difficulty accepting the catheter

Precautions:

- Observe the technical state of the moustache (that it is not obstructed).
- Fix the moustache on the head, by edge or gauze, never to the back, which causes discouragement for the patient lying down.

CHAPTER 5: COMMUNICATION

Communication is the transmission of information from one subject to another, it is the act of communicating as a process through which ideas are transmitted in order to inform, to modify behaviors.

There are elements that influence this process such as noise, context and filters.

In health care, professional work includes the establishment of direct interpersonal relationships, which go beyond the simple interaction between two individuals. The therapeutic relationship that is created between nurse and patient implies the establishment of common objectives, collaborative relationships and the exchange of mutual help, from a holistic perception.

Since the beginning of Florence Nightingale Nursing, the importance and need for communication in the relationship nurse-patient, years later H Pepla u consider communication as the method of nursing. And in the same way both Dorothea Orem and Virginia Henderson developed their theory in some way with the psychosocial sphere and proposed the development and personal relationships involving the communicative influence. The objective of communication is the transmission of a message between sender and receiver and that both share a meaning. The health personnel must know how to listen in order to understand the patient, so obtaining an optimal communication means an improvement in the quality of life and satisfaction of both the patients and their families.

Language characterizes the human being so it is impossible not to communicate. The elements that make up the communicative act are different as they are:

- Message: It is what the sender intends to convey to the receiver
- Sender: The person who chooses the message he wants to communicate.
- Receiver: The person who deciphers, decodes the message and offers an answer.
- Channel: The medium through which the message is received where great importance is given to the sense organs.
- Transmitter: It is the form that the message is transmitted, it can be written, oral,

visual, auditory.

There are many ways to establish communication, the verbal is the most common is that the person consents to choose the words that depends on cultural and social characteristics, but it is also important what is transmitted, not only with words but with gestures, expressions and where observation takes a prominent role, 80% of communication involves body movements, gestures and physical appearance. In our profession it is not only to observe the signs and symptoms but also to recognize the response to our actions.

 The current culture of care and the integration of user satisfaction in the health system, affects our responsibility as professionals to improve quality. This implies a real change in the meaning of care and quality of care.

5.1 Factors that distort communication

The interruption of the communicative process brings with it the achievement or not of the proposed objectives

- Ability to communicate. Nursing staff should have clear, simple language, low tone and soft.
- Perceptions: Respect the perceptions of the individual, family and community.
- Personal space: Perform each task in the appropriate place and time without improvisation that may affect the communicative process.
- The territoriality: The professional of the infirmary must be located in time, space and have tact at the moment of making the communicative process since the territoriality where the process is executed can intervene positively and negatively.
- Functions and relationships: If the functions attributed to each person are not fully fulfilled and if the relationships are broken for any reason from the first impact, it can bring about irreversible damage to the communicative process
- Time: It must be planned, not to exceed that the communicative process becomes an exhausting space

- The environment: Maintaining a balanced environment helps the understanding and development of the communicative process.

- Emotions and self-esteem. The psychological aspect influences both positively and negatively in the communicative process, so the nursing staff must incorporate the knowledge acquired in medical psychology to avoid damages to the patients and that contribute to frustrate the communicative process and with it the rupture, loss or deviation of the proposed objectives.

Influence of patient nursing communication in rehabilitation

Communication, when the objectives established for it are fulfilled, constitutes an important element in therapeutic support. Therefore, nursing personnel require training in communication skills so that their activity is closely related to emotional accompaniment and coping possibilities, it is important to point out the attitudes of trust as a key aspect in the nursing patient relationship ,the harmonious solidary climate, use of affordable language, taking into account the information needs of the families devoting enough time and using a protocol of care agreed upon by the professional team makes the communication effective and therefore provides a tool for the improvement in the quality of care.

Communication with the family

Nursing staff in their communication with the family focuses on equipping families with the social skills necessary for them to establish adequate and effective communication, they must be trained in patient care. When the family is notified of bad news, it often reacts with stupor and denial. This has a great impact on the family and the disease becomes the focus of activity for all members. Open communication between the health team and the family facilitates the process by which they adapt to different family events and are given the opportunity for family participation in the care of the patient.

Nurse communication with the family should meet the following criteria:

➢ Provide clear information to families about the disease and where to go.

➢ Provide assurance that the patient is receiving the care they need at each stage.

➢ Involve them in the care of the patient.

➢ Offer emotional and physical psychological support.

➢ To accompany in the agony stage and in the mourning.

➢ The professional must always adopt a helpful posture.

➢ You must take care of verbal and non-verbal language

➢ Avoid showing haste in conversations.

➢ The verbal message must be clear, avoiding ambiguity

The communication of the nursing professional with the patient.

➢ Communicate to the patient what you are, what you do, and who the members are.

➢ Recognize the patient by name and know how they prefer to be called.

➢ Being close to the patient, giving confidence.

➢ Make eye contact.

5.2 Health communication techniques

Technical communication is the process of transmitting technical information through writing, speaking, and other means of communication to a specific audience.

• Talk: It consists of a brief conference where specific topics are presented.
Advantages of the talk.

• It is economic because for its execution it is enough with the one that exposes it.

• It requires little time.

• You are bequeathing to many people at the same time.

• Later meetings can follow.

Disadvantages

• It is not suitable for changing negative habits and attitudes, since the subjects who listen remain passive, purely receptive.

The talk should not be abused because it can appear tired and the population loses interest, its use is recommended in the promotion and prevention of health, plays an important role in the health emergency, is useful for a rumor that is limiting appropriate attitudes towards population health.

Demonstration

It is a technique where action and word are combined. The one who executes the action at the same time explains. It is efficient because it is an audio-visual way, you get a dynamic vision and it creates motivation.

The panel

A group of people presents a topic in front of an audience that then participates with questions and answers.

This technique is most appropriate for prevention, recovery and rehabilitation of health.

Round Table

It differs from the panel in that the level reached by science on the subject to be discussed does not allow for agreement

This technique is recommended to be used preferably in prevention, recovery and rehabilitation.

The interview.

Planned conversation can be individual or group. It

has 3 main objectives

- Collect information
- Providing information
- Modify negative attitudes that preach health. Group dynamics

It is a dynamic process where topics, tasks and opinions are collectively analyzed and suggestions are discussed. This discussion makes each member aware of his or her own limitations, stereotypes and prejudices.

CHAPTER 6: COMMUNITY HEALTH PROMOTION AND PREVENTION

The phenomenon of providing care is as old as the beginning of life. Care is innate in the human being; man, like all living beings, has always had the need to care, to maintain the continuity of life and of course to do so in a conscious way and oriented to human welfare.

By combining knowledge and care, but neither can be dispensed with. Governments spend most of thei r health budgets on healing and rehabilitating people, ignoring the value of health education, which sets the tone for maintaining health and knowledge of healthy actions to maintain it. Therefore, the training of health professionals must be instructed in the transmission of knowledge in the communities and during their training process, offer them the necessary tools to be able to raise the quality of life of the inhabitants in the communities and work on the basis of prevention in health issues. Therefore, the preparation of the citizens is needed in a country where the citizens carry out tasks with quality of excelection, it is a prepared nation. A society is prepared when all or most of its citizens are; an individual is prepared when he or she can face the problems that arise in the workplace and solve them. In this way, the concept of preparation expresses the problem, the starting point of pedagogical science and its category.

Nursing is considered the art of caring, a profession endowed with a body of knowledge that makes it possible for the professionals in this career to offer intelligent care. Therefore, one must learn how to educate so that this care fulfills the expected objective. For it, the professional of infirmary must have an integral multidisciplinary formation, be formed with pedagogical an d didactic bases notions the philosophy, sociology, psychology, anthropology, ethics, bioethics, basic sciences of foundation and the own contents of the discipline of infirmary if they will be able to develop the educative competition with an integral approach, of resolution of situations and problems that will make the effectiveness of the action. This requires a reflective and comprehensive effort and the development of applied models that make the best interpretation of the task possible. The education in the process of formation of the person, must be adapted to these essential characteristics. Every person has the right to reach his or her maximum development or self-realization . The psychological perspective analyzes the dynamics of individuals, as well a s their qualitative characteristics, in the various dimensions of the person: inheritance, specific abilities, attitudes, interests an d values, and individual and socia lbehavior. The p e c t i v a p e d a g o g y o f i n d i v i d u a l i n d i v i d u a l i n d e v e l o p m e n t a n d p r o j e c t i o n a l i n t e r v e l o p m e n t a t i o n a l s o c i a l a n d p r o j e c t i o n a l p r o g r a m m e n t s a n d d d e v e l o p m e n t proposals. This p r i n c i p l e is c a l l e d individualized teaching and it is the set of methods and techniques that allow acting simultaneously on several people, adapting the work to the development of their aptitudes and development.

Florence N i g h t i n g a l e began research in nursing and was the first to write about the discipline. Since that time, nursing has been a way of providing care and educating people to maintain their health in the best possible conditions.

6.1 Nursing fields of action in health education

The fields of action of e n f e r m e r i a affect all the processes of Health, providing in each one of them education for the s a l u d , being this a situation to attend in the process of professional formation of the nurse.

Health education is one of the activities carried out by nurses, an activity they learn d u r i n g their careers. And that is done, indispensable in the act of taking care of the health and the life of the people. With the beginning of the world or

Christianity has given rise to the humanitarian approach of the citizens. In the c o n t r a

The reform continues this r e f e r e n c e, to be carried out by loyal orders such as the Daughters of Charity, whose w o r k of c a r i n g for sick p e o p l e, left two principles alive, day and night, in Primary Care nurses:

In general, the activity of nursing emerges as something primitive but inherent to the human quality of the women who exercised it and in doing so, began to exercise a relationship of interdependence with the person was the subject of care, where as can

39

be seen   , the transfer of knowledge for the conservation of health began, thus initiating the educational processes of care towards the person who received the care. Later, th e foundation   for   professional nursing wa   s laid when Florence Nightingale, in her Nursing Notes (1998) attempted   finalize the specific application of nursing to health care. In the theoretical development of nursing, concepts and propositions are considered that raise the relations between those **who** have been called meta paradigms. The meta-paradigmatic concepts that make up the conceptual framework of e n f e r m e r y and that are present in all nursing models, such as the models of Orem, Henderson, Roy, Rogers, Johnson, King and Levine, are The person, health, environment and nursing care.

CHAPTER 7: SYNTHESIS OF NURSING THEORIES AND MODELS APPLIED IN COMMUNITY CARE

Nursing is also a profession with a university degree that is dedicated to the integral care of the individual, the family and the community in all stages of the life cycle and in its development processes. In Spain and Colombia, there is another oficio within the Nursing profession whose functions complement the work of nurses: the qualified technician in nursing auxiliary care, better known as a nursing assistant.

The modelsand theories of Nursing aim to describe, establish and examine the phenomena that make up the practice of GeneralNursing.

It is assumed by the discipline that in order to determine that a nursing theory exists it must contain the elements of the nursing meta-paradigm.

Each discipline makes its own the terms related to the theory and its development with the fin to provide it with a body of knowledge that allows it toguide the exercise of the discipline.

7.1 Types of models

Each author groups the models according to their own criteria. It is usually based on the role that nursing plays in providing care. Thus, we can divide them into:

• Naturalistic models.

• Models of substitution or assistance.

•Interrelationship

models. Naturalistic

models

Its main representative is Florence Nightingale. In 1859 she discusses definir the nature of nursing care in her book Notes on Nursing;

"There is a tendency to believe that medicine cures. Nothing is less true, medicine is surgery of functions as true surgery is surgery of organs, neither one nor the other cures, only nature can cure.

- What nursing care does in both cases is to put the patient in his or her best health.

7.2 Florence Nightingale's Theory

He had understood the need to have a reference scheme, a conceptual framework. From this first attempt at conceptualization, until this question is again formally asked, almost a century goes by. It is the simplest of all the models, where he stated that nursing knowledge was very different from medical science knowledge and he made clear the role of the nurse

I point out that one of the results of nursing is to conserve the patient's vital energy. I propose that cleanliness, ventilation and food are indispensable elements for the recovery of the patient and I define a concept of health in a state of well-being that translates into taking advantage of people's energies.

Models of substitution or assistance

The role of nursing consists of supplying or helping to carry out the actions that the person cannot carry out in a moment of his life, actions that preserve life, encouraging both the self-care of the person.

The two most important representatives of this trend are Virginia Hendersonand Dorothea Orem.

Interrelationship Models

In these models the role of the nurse is to encourage the adaptation of the person in a changing environment, promoting either interpersonal (nurse-patient) or patient relations with their environment.

The most representative models are those of HildegardePeplau-, CallistaRoy, MarthaE. Rogersand Myra Levine.

7.3 Virginia Henderson Model

Theoretical basis

- It is a model ofsubstitutionorhelp.
- Part of Maslow's concept of human needs

the human being is a biopsychosocialbeingwith needs that he tries to cover independently according to his habits, culture, etc. The human being has 14 basic needs:

Breathing, eating and drinking, evacuating, moving and maintaining posture, sleeping and resting, dressing and undressing, maintaining body temperature, keeping clean, avoiding dangers, communicating, offering worship, working, playing and learning.

Healthis the ability of a person to perform all those activities that allow him/her to keep basic needs satisfied.

The human being must also be seen from a

biopsychosocial, spiritual and holistic perspective, different in their feelings and emotions. The overload of work in the hospital units makes this care as such increasingly difficult. Let us remember that those of us who offer our nursing services do not make value judgments, we empathize. and we accompany them to the last breath.

Methodology of care

It consists of a plan of care: a problem-solving process. The human being should be seen from a biopsychosocial, spiritual and holistic perspective, different in his feelings and emotions. The overload of work in the hospital units makes it more and more difficult to be a patient. Let us remember that those who offer our nursing services do not make value judgments, and we accompany them until the last breath.

7.4 M o d e l o f Dorothea Orem

Theoretical basis

- It is a model ofsubstitutionorhelp.
  - Maslow's theory of human needs
  - Generalsystemstheory.P

resumptions and values

For Dorothea Orem the human being is a biological, psychological organism, and in interaction with its environment, to which it is subjected. It has the capacity to create, communicate and carry out activities beneficiosas for itself and for others.

Healthis a state that significa structural and functional integrity that is achieved through universal actions called self-care I conceptualize the proper role of the nurse in caring for the healthy and sick person in their activities to contribute to their health or recovery I declare that the performance of nursing depends on the doctor and that human beings have basic needs that must be met and are normally covered by the healthy individual.

Self-careis a human need that constitutes every action that a human being performs through his values, beliefs, etc. with the fin to maintain life, health and well-being. These are deliberate actions that require learning. When the person cannot carry out these actions by himself, either because of limitation or disability, a situation of dependence on self-care is produced.

There are three types of self-care:

Those derived from the fundamental needs that each individual has: eating, drinking, breathing, ...

Those derived from the needs específicas that arise in certain moments of development vi such as: childhood, adolescence, adulthood and old age.

7.5 Peplau Model

Model established by nurse HildegardPeplau

Theoretical basis

- Model of interrelationship.

- Psychoanalytic theory.

- Theory of human needs

- Concept of motivation.

- Concept of personal development.

- Orientation phase. The patient tries clarificar his dificultades and the extent of the help needs. The nurse assesses the person's situation

- Phase of identificación. The patient clarifica his situation, identifica the need for help and responds to people who offer help. The nurse diagnoses the situation and formulates the plan ofcare.

- Exploitation phase. The patient makes use of the nursing services and gets the most out of them. The nurse implements the careplan, helping the person and him or herself to grow into maturity

- Resolution phase. The patient resumes his independence. The nurse evaluatesthe growth that has occurred between the two.

Nursing functions: In Hildegarde Peplau's model, they consist of helping the human being to mature personally by facilitating a creative, constructive and productive life.

7.6 Callista Roy Model

Methodology of care

Nursing care process.Callista Roy's Model Adaptation Theory

Presumptions and values: The human being is a biopsychosocial being - in constant interaction with the environment. This inter-action is carried out by means of adaptation which, for Roy, consists of the adaptation of the 4 spheres of life:

- Area fisiológica. Circulation, temperature, oxygen, liquids, sleep, activity, feeding and elimination.

- Area of self-image. The image one has of oneself.

- Role domain area. The different roles that a human being plays throughout his life.

- Area of independence. Positive interactions with his environment, in this case, the people with whom he exchanges influencias that provide him with a balance of his self-image and mastery of roles.

The human being, in turn, is at a certain point in what he calls the

"continuum" (or path) health-illness. This point can be closer to health or disease by virtue of each individual's ability to respond to the stimuli they receive from their environment. If he responds positively, adapting, he will approach the state of health, if not, he will become ill.

Health is a state and process of being and becomes integrated and global. This can be seen at modificada by the stimuli of the environment, which for Callista are

- Focal stimuli. Precipitate changes to be faced. For example, a flu process.

- Contextual stimuli. All those who are present in the process. For example, room temperature.

- Residual stimuli. These are the values and beliefs from past experiences, which may have influencia in the present situation. For example, shelter, home

46

treatments.

7.7 Martha Rogers' model

Theoretical basis
- Model of interrelationship.

- General systems theory

- Evolutionary theory.

Presumptions and values: The human being is a whole unificado in constant relation with his environment, with which he exchanges matter and energy; and that he differs from the rest of the living beings by his capacity to change this environment and to make choices that allow him to develop as a person.

For Rogers, the human being is an energy field interacting with another energy field: the environment. This is evident in the principles of thermodynamics, on which his theoretical framework is based. The flujo constant of waves between people and the environment are the basis of nursing activities. Life is a flujo of experiences. To be alive is to become irreversibly more complex, diverse and differentiated - nothing is ever what it used to be. The capacity to do, describes the way in which beings interact with their environment to update their potentials that allow them to develop and participate, therefore, in the creation of human and environmental reality.

Health is the constant harmonic maintenance of the human being with his environment. If harmony is broken, health and well-being disappear.

Nursing Functions In this model, the individual is expected to reach his/her maximum health potential.

CHAPTER 8: ACCIDENTS IN THE HOME

The word Accident has a Latin origin, accident, which means chance. The WHO considers that the accident is a fortuitous event generally unpleasant or harmful, independent of human will, caused by an external force that acts quickly and is manifested by the appearance of organic injuries or mental disorders. They constitute the fifth cause of death in the world.

Domestic accidents are those that occur in the home itself, patios, gardens, garages, access floors, stairwells. All places belonging to the home. It is in the home, where the family usually spends most of its time throughout its life, and it is there where there is a possibility of a domestic accident of any kind. Although all the members of the family have the same possibilities of suffering an accident, it is the children and the elderly who suffer most frequently. Their age and their situation in life make them the most helpless and vulnerable because of their ignorance, carelessness, weakness and mental characteristics.

8.1 Most common accidents

The statistics of victims of accidents increase every year, behaving as the first causes of death worldwide, many of them being avoidable and preventable. In the reviews carried out the main causes of accidents at different ages are

- Falls
- Wounds
- Burns
- Ingestion of toxic substances
- Choking
- Electrocution

8.2 General causes

Carrying out a causal analysis of the appearance of the accidents, general elements are found that make the appearance or occurrence of the accidents possible, such as

- Poor lighting
- Wet, wet and slippery floors
- Very high or narrow steps
- Running down the stairs
- Climbing on chairs or other objects
- High beds
- Poisoning with liquids and powders
- Electrical Cables
- Carpets
- Inadequate handling of household appliances
- Fire by candles
- Gas emergency.
- Concave baths
- Containers with water where a small child can immerse himself.
- Plants with small fruits that can ingest or introduce and holes.
- Poorly plugged wells
  Most frequent causes in children
- Cradle
- Bed
- Bathroom
- Dining room
- Street
- Field
  Most common causes in older adults
- Falls
- Wounds

- Fractures

The risk of the elderly is over added since the use of psycho-pharmaceuticals or other CNS depressants and osteomyoarticular conditions, visual deficit and balance disorders led to the precipitation of accidents, in addition to structural problems of housing and the presence of objects on the floor. Most older adults have little knowledge about the causes of accidents, much less the behavior to follow when faced with an event.

It is important to mention the dangers that technology exerts and that can cause physical and emotional damage in some stages of life by submerging them in diseases such as depression, anxiety and low self-esteem because it does not allow the development of the necessary skills to demonstrate the qualities and tools that each one has.

We also have biological hazards of food origin such as bacteria, viruses and parasites. These organisms are often associated with contaminated handlers and raw products that are accidentally introduced to humans.

8.3 Activities to prevent accidents in the home

The nurse in his community intervention being known the main causes of the appearance of the accidents, will carry out an action plan where it involves activities of easy understanding by the inhabitants of the community in his charge and that help to raise the perception of the risk in the houses and surroundings and contribute to the reduction of the accidents. We can mention some of them.

1. Keep small objects and toys out of reach that can get into the mouth or nose and cause choking.
2. Cutting food into small pieces and having adults supervise this process.
3. Do not neglect your baby when he is breastfeeding
4. Avoid the child's play with plastic bags.

Inside the house
1 Test an evacuation plan in case of fire.

2 Place locks on cabinets, to prevent children from accessing harmful substances

3 Keep electrical cables out of the reach of children

4 Place plates on the outlets to avoid being electrocuted.

5 Keep hazardous chemicals out of reach of children and heat sources

6 Do not use soft drink containers to store toxic substances

7 Prepare cabinet for medications out of reach of children

8 Place accessories on doors that prevent them from closing suddenly.

9 No stairs without handrails.

10 Use carpets in the bathroom to avoid slipping

11 In the case of an older adult, have a lamp near the bed to light when getting up.

12 The use of the cane in the elderly.

13 Keep objects such as knives, scissor needles, etc., in a safe place.

14 If you have to make physical efforts, you must do it with bent knees, straight back and feet slightly separated to avoid tears or muscular contractions.

15 Avoid children's playground in the kitchen 16 Keep

the griddle out of reach of children

17 Place safety gates at the top and bottom of the stairs

18 Have identified in your home the points of risk that can cause an accident in order to reduce them.

8.4 Action of the community health professional in the prevention of accidents

Nursing as a profession encompasses the care of a society and its relationship with its environment where the conditions that surround it are taken into account for the formulation of strategies according to the identified needs.

The clinical community, administrative environment has become a virtuous circle where the nurse has exercised his or her knowledge achieving to highlight personal care as a differential factor in the execution of daily activities.

Strengthening community nursing practices in order to reduce the occurrence of accidents are social objectives and the challenges that arise in community nursing is fundamental to nursing care. The community nurse must promote programs for the prevention of accidents in the home allowing their work to increase the levels of knowledge of caregivers and promote actions aimed at obtaining a safer environment, assess the impact and reduction of potential hazards of accidents in families and thus raise the quality of life of their dependents in the community. Considering that the main medicine is prevention, health promotion actions in primary health care must be strengthened, the nurse with community charge must carry out a multidisciplinary and intersectoral work in order to guarantee a healthy environment without risks of accidents and with them to achieve a healthy community. The responsibilities of the professional of the infirmary are immersed in the pedagogical assistential administrative activities where several tools are implemented that help to provide the action proposed in each case.

From a wide perspective, the profession of nursing applied in a community environment is supported by the WHO through the strategy created for the conservation of healthy environments where the theoretical, axiological and moral bases of the profession are based, making it a fundamental link of the global chain of interactions to communities that strengthens the functioning of health systems. Nursing professionals within the health and safety field apply knowledge and tools within the community in order to promote, maintain and improve the health of the population. Leadership in this discipline makes it possible to direct and coordinate the different processes or health plans in any environment such as the community.

Nursing Staff Tools

➢ Instrumental: The use of the Nursing Care Process, the perfect tool for planning care that impacts the health of the individual, family and community.
➢ Personal: In the management implemented by the nursing professional: listening, active is a tool for attending and understanding the subject of care, establishing a relationship of trust that leads to the creation of care and risk prevention habits.

- ➢ Systematic: The innate leadership of the nurse provides adaptive characteristics to different environments to achieve the design of programs for an improvement in the community environment promoting family bonding guiding families in the adoption of good practices.
- ➢ Specific: Relating the theories and skills of the nurse, structured care plans are generated through a methodology under the concepts of the profession which are unique and indispensable to achieve the proposed objectives.

These nursing tools allow the achievement of care goals where some Nursing theorists like Orem, Watson, and Lenninger are used in the management process and that through the implementation of the Meta Paradigm: person, environment, health and nursing, the nursing care process is involved achieving the care needs of individuals, families and communities

The nurse must empower and visualize her managerial role within the communities

In this way it can have greater relevance within the different social groups and also facilitates better management in dealing with tasks, crises and situations that arise in the community.

The nexus of nursing leadership must be networked so that it can be demonstrated that professionals are in constant interaction. The community work is focused on health promotion by achieving teamwork, innate roles, interpersonal relationships, the subject of care with the interaction in the community and families, achieving the generation of knowledge through health education and risk prevention which are impacted by the tools already mentioned.

BIBLIOGRAPHY

1. Attention to the elderly. SemFYC Elderly Working Group, Ediciones Eurobook, SL. Madrid 1997:11-47.

2. C. De Alba Romero, J. M. Baena Díez, M. C. de Hoyos Alonso, A. Gorroñogoitia Iturbe, C. Litargo Gil, L. Martín.

3. Muñoz, A ECS De la promoción de la salud a los ambientes de trabajo saludables, Salud de los Trabajadores 18(2) 141-152 [Online]; 2010 [cited 2019, Available from: http://wwwscieloorgve/scielophp?script=sci_ar

4. Torres C, Perception of the quality of nursing care in hospitalized oncology patients Cuidadte magazine 2(2) 138-148 [Online]; 2011 Available from: https://wwwrevistacuidarteorg/indexphp/cuidarte/article/view/49/688.

5. Delgado A, The Nursing Care Act as a Foundation for Professional and Research Advances in Nursing 33(3) 412-419 [Online]; 2015, Available from:https://searchproquestcom/docview/1819126028?accountid=47900

6. Muñoz, A ECS De la promoción de la salud a los ambientes de trabajo saludables, Salud de los Trabajadores 18(2) 141-152 [Online]; 2010 [cited 2019, Available from: http://wwwscieloorgve/scielophp?script=sci_ar

7. Torres C, Perception of the quality of nursing care in hospitalized oncology patients Cuidadte magazine 2(2) 138-148 [Online]; 2011 Available from: https://wwwrevistacuidarteorg/indexphp/cuidarte/article/view/49/688

8. Vega F Ramírez, The role of communication campaigns in health promotion and injury prevention in occupational health1(2)137-154 Recovered 12 July2018 [Online];2010Available from: http://wwwaecses/1_2_comunicacion%20salud%20laboralpdf.

9. According to the PalmaF , the work of the Nursing: literature review Science and Nursing 21(2) 11-20 [Online]; 2015, Available from: https://scieloconicytcl/scielophp?pid=S0717-95532015000200002&script=sci_arttext.

10. Tokur M, Using the Omaha System in Occupational Health Nursing

Applications: Advantages of a Common Language in the Diagnosis Intervention and Evaluation of Nurses Health Problems Revista Elsevier Volume 152 (7) 488-494   [Online];   2014Available
from:
https://wwwsciencedirectcom/science/article/pii/S1877042814053051

11. Bathrobe Mancera, D.M. (2009). The importance of transculturality in nursing knowledge. Rev Paraninfo Digital, 3 (7), Available at:
</para/n7/100d. php>. Consulted on January 24, 2014.

12. Artigas Lelong, B., Vennasar Veny, M. (2009). Health in the 21st century: the challenge of multicultural care.

13. González Juárez, L., Noreña Peña, A.L. (2011). Intercultural communication as a means to promote culturally acceptable care. Rev ENEO-UNAM, 8(1), 55-60.

14. Benavides M. Avoidable accidents: Children's injuries and their relationships with social and family environments. Space for Children 2012; 18:29-31.

15. Bustos E, Cabrales G, Cerón M, Naranjo Y. Epidemiology of accidental injuries in children: Review of international and national statistics. Bol Med Hosp Infant Mex 2014; 71(2):68-75.

16. Gorrita RR, Barrientos G, Gorrita Y. Risk factors, family functioning and unintentional injuries in children under five. Journal of Medical Sciences of Havana 2016; 22(1):42-57.

17. Martínez M, Gutiérrez H, Alonso M, Hernández L. Knowledge of a group of mothers about the prevention of accidents in the home. Re-view of Medical Sciences of Havana 2015; 21(2):335-345.

18. Cedrés A, Morosini F, Margni C, López A, Alegretti M, Dall'Orso P, et al. Animal bites in children. What is the current situation in the Pediatric?

19. Emergency Department at Pereira Rossell Hospital? Arch Pediatr Urug 2018; 89(1):15-20. DOI: http://dx.doi.org/10.31134/ap.89.1.3.

20. Garzón N. Unintentional injuries a public health problem. Bogotá D.C: National Institute of Legal Medicine; 2015.

21. Torres M. Fonseca C, Díaz Martínez M, del Campo O, Roché R. Accidents in childhood: A current problem in pediatrics. MEDISAN 2010.

22. Cardero E, Mojena G, Porto Y, del Río L, Calas G. Clinical therapeutic characterization of children and adolescents with Aero digestive foreign bodies. MEDISAN 2018; 22(4):384-393.

23. Olmedo M.C.; Systematic for the protocolization of nursing care. Journal of Quality Care (online). 2010. (May 02, 2012); No.25.

24. Colliére MF. Promoting life. Mexico: Mc Graw-Hill In- teramericana; 1993.

25. Ministry of Health. Interinstitutional Commission of Nursing. Evaluation of the quality of nursing services, 2002.

26. Peña K, Rodríguez J. Nursing in the face of chaos and complexity Culture of care. 2003; 14:79-82.

27. Collective of authors, Family and Social Nursing, Chapters 18. Editorial Ciencias Médicas de la Habana, Cuba 2004.

28. Álvarez Sintes, Topics of General Integral Medicine, Volume II, Chapter 15. Medical Sciences Publishing House of Havana, Cuba 2001.

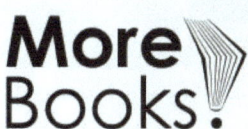
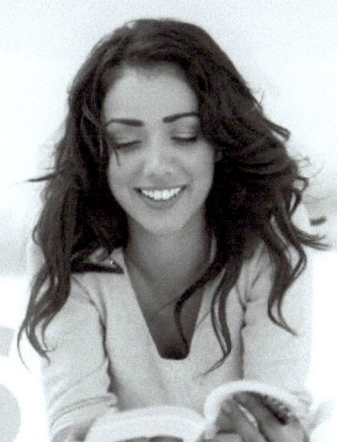

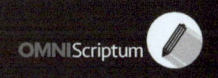

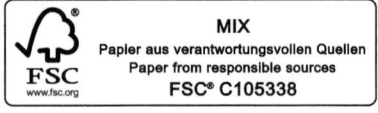
Printed by Books on Demand GmbH, Norderstedt / Germany